GERD COOKBOOK FOR SENIORS 2024

Flavorful Healing a Senior's Guide to GERD-Friendly Cooking

Magdalene Charles

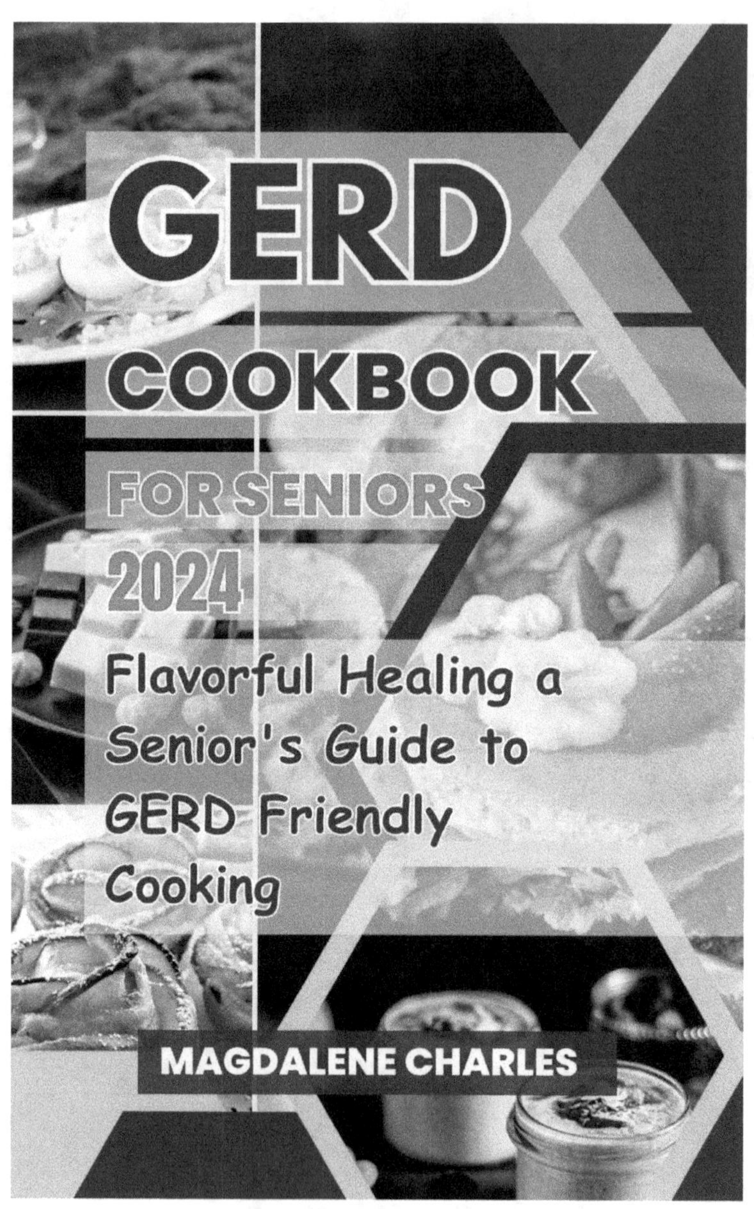

GERD
COOKBOOK
FOR SENIORS
2024
Flavorful Healing a
Senior's Guide to
GERD Friendly
Cooking
MAGDALENE CHARLES

TABLE OF CONTENT

OVERVIEW

Begin your journey to digestive wellness with "Flavorful Healing: A Senior's Guide to GERD-Friendly Cooking," your culinary companion. With the health of older citizens in mind, this cookbook offers a delectable road map for overcoming the difficulties associated with gastroesophageal reflux disease (GERD).

You will find a symphony of flavors on these pages that are intended to calm and nourish, along with a wide variety of recipes that are adapted to suit the dietary needs of people with GERD. We recognize how important it is to be able to enjoy meals without having to deal with heartburn, and this cookbook is devoted to making eating enjoyable again.

Our strategy embraces the wealth of healthful, senior-friendly components that improve taste and health rather than focusing just on limitations. Every recipe has been carefully chosen to achieve a harmonious blend of flavor and digestibility, so you can enjoy every bite without sacrificing nutrients or flavor.

"Flavorful Healing" offers detailed directions, practical advice, and a wide range of delectable options, from breakfast treats to cozy dinners and all in between, regardless of your level of culinary experience. Our mission is to equip you with the information and resources you need to prepare meals that not only satisfy your palate but also adhere to GERD standards.

Together, let's celebrate the happiness that comes with eating well and feeling well as we set off on our gastronomic expedition. For seniors in 2024 and beyond, here's to tasty recovery and a revitalized sense of culinary delight.

CHAPTER 1

RECIPES FOR BREAKFAST

Maple syrup pancakes

Ingredients:
- Butter 25 g
- flour 125 g
- Medium eggs 2
- Fresh whole milk 200 g
- Baking powder for cakes 6 g
- Brown sugar 15 g

TO SEAL:
- Maple syrup to taste

Instructions

The first step in making pancakes is to melt the butter over low heat and allow it to cool. Separate the egg whites and yolks in the meanwhile. Transfer the yolks into a bowl and use a hand whisk to beat them. Next, add the room-temperature melted butter and the flushed milk, continuing to whisk. Mix the blend until it turns transparent. Whisk to integrate after adding the yeast to the flour and sifting everything into the dish containing the egg mixture.

Now, slowly add the sugar to the egg whites that you set aside, beating them until they are white and foamy. Be careful not to disassemble them by adding the egg whites to the mixture from top to bottom.

Warm a large nonstick pan (ideally with a thick bottom) over medium heat (not high; otherwise, you won't give the dough enough time to rise well during cooking, and the pancakes will turn too dark). If needed, grease the pan with a little butter, spreading it over the surface with the aid of kitchen paper. You don't need to spread the preparation when you pour a ladleful into the middle of the saucepan. The pancake is finished when bubbles start to form on the surface and the base turns golden. Use a spatula to flip it over to the other side, just like you would with an omelet or crepe, and brown the other side as well. Once you've finished the remaining dough, stack the pancakes one on top of the other and gradually arrange them on a serving platter. With these dosages, about 12 pancakes should form. Serve them warm with a maple syrup sprinkle on top. You can serve the pancakes with sugar or fresh fruit according to your preference.

Muffin with chocolate drops

Ingredients:
- Softened butter at room temperature 125 g
- 00 flour 265 g
- Sugar 135 g
- Whole milk at room temperature 135 g
- Eggs (about 2) at room temperature 110 g
- Dark chocolate drops 100 g
- Vanilla bean 1
- Satin bicarbonate 1 tsp

- Salt up to a pinch
- Baking powder 1

Instructions

- To get the chocolate chip muffins ready Stir with the electric whisk butter, which had been allowed to soften for at least an hour at room temperature, and the sugar, until a creamy and foamy combination was achieved. Next, chop a vanilla bean and use the knife's back to scrape the seeds. Transfer the latter to the basin containing the sugar and butter. Restart the whips and gradually add the room-temperature eggs one at a time so that the components don't come loose. Now immediately sift the flour, baking soda, and baking powder into the basin containing the mixture. Incorporate the powders by operating the whisk again and adding a pinch of salt. Once the dough starts to become more uniform, thin it out with room-temperature milk and pour it flush. The mixture will be soft and compact at this point.

- Using a spatula, stir in the 80 grams of chocolate chips to fully include them. Next, pour the mixture into a disposable bag without a nozzle. If this isn't possible, you can also use a spoon for a cleaner finish. With less than an inch separating the bottom, fill the paper cups two thirds of the way to the top in a muffin pan. The weight of each muffin must be around 70 grams. Drizzle the leftover 20 drops of chocolate over the cupcakes and bake in a preheated 180°F static oven for 18–20 minutes (if the oven is ventilated, bake at 160°F for 13–15 minutes). Your chocolate chip muffins are now prepared for consumption.

Yoghurt plum cake

Ingredients:

- 00 flour 300 g
- Eggs (about 5) 300 g
- Butter 200 g
- Icing sugar 200 g
- Low-fat yogurt 150 g
- Potato starch 50 g
- Baking powder for sweets 15 g
- Vanilla bean seeds 1
- Salt up to 4 g

FOR MOLDS

- Butter to taste
- 00 flour to taste

Instructions

- Prepare the yogurt plumcake by putting together a mixer with large, reasonably powerful blades. Put the cubed butter, vanilla bean seeds, eggs, flour, yogurt, icing sugar, salt, yeast, and starch in the container. For roughly four minutes, work at your fastest pace. Grease and flour two 16 x 8 cm molds that are slightly flared in the meantime. Once the mixture is uniformly distributed, pour it into the molds. Now dip a knife blade into the melted butter and then into the middle of each of the two plum cakes. This will guarantee consistent cooking growth.

- Place the plum cakes in a static oven that has been warmed. They must cook in two stages: for 15 minutes at 185 °C and then for 30 minutes at 165 °C.
- Remove from the oven as soon as cooked, and allow to cool fully. Now that they are exposed and dusted with icing sugar, your yogurt plum cakes are prepared for tasting.

Vegetable tart

Ingredients:

- 1 pack of puff pastry of about 300 g
- 2 courgettes
- 4 potatoes
- 4 eggs
- 30 g of grated cheese
- basil
- chives
- extra virgin olive oil
- Salt

Instructions

- Cut the courgettes into pieces in preparation for the veggie tart. Slice the courgettes into pieces that are roughly 5 mm thick after cutting off both ends. After lightly salting them, set them aside to drain in a colander. After peeling, washing, and drying the potatoes, chop them and place them in a skillet with two teaspoons of heating oil, much like you would for fried chips. After browning, simmer the potatoes for ten minutes. Take them off the burner and place them on paper towels.

- After the zucchini has thoroughly dried, put it in the same pan and cook it for 15 minutes, stirring it frequently. Beat the eggs in the interim. After cooking, place the zucchini and potatoes in a bowl, then stir in the beaten eggs, grated cheese, chopped and salted chives, and basil. Place the puff pastry in an oil-greased tart pan. Evenly distribute the prepared filling, then bake for approximately 25 minutes at 200° in a preheated oven. After letting the vegetable tart sit for roughly ten minutes, proceed to serve it.

Potato omelette

Ingredients:

- Eggs 6
- Potatoes 500 g

- Parmesan cheese 100 g
- Parsley to taste
- Salt to taste
- Seed oil to taste

Instructions

- Before preparing the potato omelet, fill a pan with water and bring it to a boil. Peel and cut the potatoes in the interim. Let the potatoes boil for around five minutes. finely chopped parsley to add to the potatoes while they cook. Now combine the eggs, grated cheese, minced parsley, and salt in a bowl. Mix the ingredients together at this point. After the potatoes are cooked through, drain and allow to cool before adding them to the egg mixture.
- Cooking now involves heating a drizzle of seed oil in a skillet and adding the mixture once it's hot. Cook for fifteen minutes over medium heat with the lid on, occasionally rotating

the pan. Flip the omelet over the lid and quickly and decisively turn the pan upside down when the top is still moist but not extremely soft. Return the omelet to the pan to cook the other side, replace the lid, and cook for a further five minutes. The omelet will be ready after this. It can be served either hot or cold.

Apple muffin

Ingredients:
- Apples 310 g
- 00 flour 300 g
- Greek yogurt 150 g
- Sugar 120 g
- Eggs (about 4) 220 g
- Baking powder for sweets 16 g
- Lemon zest 1

Instructions
- Before preparing the potato omelet, fill a pan with water and bring it to a boil.

Peel and cut the potatoes in the interim. Let the potatoes boil for around five minutes. finely chopped parsley to add to the potatoes while they cook. Now combine the eggs, grated cheese, minced parsley, and salt in a bowl. Mix the ingredients together at this point. After the potatoes are cooked through, drain and allow to cool before adding them to the egg mixture. Cooking now involves heating a drizzle of seed oil in a skillet and adding the mixture once it's hot. Place the cover on and cook for fifteen minutes on medium heat, rotating the pan from time to time. When the surface is still damp but not particularly soft, quickly and decisively turn the omelet over the lid, flipping the pan upside down. Return the omelet to the pan to cook the other side, replace the lid, and cook for a further five minutes. The omelet will

be ready after this. It can be served
either cold or heated.

Apple muffin

Ingredients:
- Apples 310 g
- 00 flour 300 g
- Greek yogurt 150 g
- Sugar 120 g
- Eggs (about 4) 220 g
- Baking powder for sweets 16 g
- Lemon zest 1

Instructions
- The eggs should first be poured into a big basin and beaten with forks or an electric whisk. After adding the sugar gradually, beat for about five minutes. Remix the mixture with the whisk after adding the yogurt. Keeping the whisk running, sift the flour and yeast into a different bowl and add them one spoonful at a time. Lastly, stir in the

grated zest of lemon. After washing, cut the apples into wedges, and remove the peel. After chopping the wedges into cubes, add them to the dough and evenly mix them in with a spatula. Using paper cups, line a muffin pan and fill each with around two tablespoons of dough. Bake for around 25 to 28 minutes at 180 ° in a static oven that has been preheated. After cooking, remove from the oven and let it cool. You are now able to taste your apple muffins!

Baked Frittata

Ingredients:
- Eggs 8
- Grated cheese 100 g
- Chives to taste
- Thyme to taste
- Salt to taste
- Extra virgin olive oil 10 g

FOR BRUSHING AND SPREADING THE TRAY

- Extra virgin olive oil to taste
- Breadcrumbs to taste

Instructions

- To make the frittata, first coat a rectangle baking dish measuring 26 by 19 cm with oil and then line it with breadcrumbs 2. Whisk together the eggs, grated cheese, oil, and finely chopped chives. Add salt and peeled thyme next. After that, beat for a few more seconds to create a homogenous mixture.
- After transferring everything to the oven dish, bake for 25 minutes at 170 ° in a static oven that has been preheated. Serve your frittata hot out of the oven to kick off the day!

Porridge

Ingredients:
- Oat flakes 140 g
- Whole milk 220 g
- Water 200 g
- Salt to taste

TO SEAL
- Honey to taste
- Strawberries to taste
- Flaked almonds to taste

Instructions
- In order to prepare the porridge, first place the oats in a bowl, cover with water, and let soak for approximately one hour (the night before is best). Transfer the oats into the saucepan, stir in the milk and a small amount of salt, and cook, stirring frequently, for about 4–5 minutes. Turn off the heat, move the porridge to a bowl, and add honey once the oats are mushy and have absorbed the milk. Add almonds

and fresh strawberry slices as garnish.
Present your heated oatmeal.

Salted Plum Cake

Ingredients:
- 00 flour 200 g
- Eggs 3
- Raw ham 150 g
- Whole milk 150 ml
- Extra virgin olive oil 60 ml
- Salt to taste
- Instant yeast for savory preparations 1 sachet
- Grated cheese 150 g

Instructions
- Grated cheese is added to a bowl of flour and yeast mixture to make the salted plum cake. After thoroughly mixing the ingredients, add the raw ham and whisk once more. Next, pour in the flush of extra virgin olive oil.

Beat the eggs with the milk and salt in a separate basin, then pour the resulting liquid into the flour, cheese, and ham mixture. Using a spoon, stir the items until thoroughly combined. Line a one-liter plum cake mold with flour and butter, then fill it with dough. Using the back of a spoon, level it, then bake it for 45 to 50 minutes at 180 ° C. Use a toothpick to ensure it's cooked through. Once the salted plum cake is done, take it out of the mold while it's still warm and allow it to cool fully. Present your salted apple crisp!

CHAPTER 2

RECIPES FOR STARTER

Boiled eggs

Ingredients:
- 4 fresh eggs

Instructions

The first step in making hard-boiled eggs is to put the entire eggs in a large pot with cold water (the water must cover the eggs).
Next, ignite the saucepan and allow it to come to a boil. Calculate nine minutes of cooking time from the boil. To cool the eggs, take the saucepan off the heat source after nine minutes and run it under cold water. This will make it possible for you to peel them without getting scorched. After you carefully remove every shell and split the eggs in half, you'll find that the insides are properly cooked!

You can enjoy boiled eggs however you choose!

Cheese waffles

Ingredients:

- Cheese 160 grams

Instructions

Starting with the support, cut the parchment paper strips into six equal squares of around 25 cm. Then, fill each square with a heaping tablespoon of grated cheese. Spread the cheese to create a circle with a diameter of about 20 cm using the back of the spoon. Now, place each sheet in the oven (or microwave) on high for a few seconds, or until the cheese starts to melt. All ingredients should be cooked at 180° for a few minutes, or until the waffle edges start to become golden. If you stop at this point, your waffles will be round and flat; they are ready to be served once they have cooled completely. Work the pods while they are still warm and flexible to give them the shape of a "bowl." The pods are thin and easily shatter, so this is a very careful procedure. After taking a disk of cheese and its parchment paper, put it inside a square or round bowl. Press the cheese toward the bottom of the bowl with the back of a spoon to swiftly mold it into the desired form. Then, let it cool. The waffles can now be carefully taken out of the bowl, the baking paper removed, and placed aside. You can now stuff your cheese wafers with whatever filling you choose.

Gratinated prawns

Ingredients:
- Gratinated prawns
- Shrimp (about 16) 200 g
- Salt to taste
- White wine 80 ml

FOR THE PANURE

- Breadcrumbs 50 g
- Grana Padano PDO 25 g
- Extra virgin olive oil to taste
- Parsley to be chopped 10 g
- Salt to taste

Instructions

To begin cleaning the shellfish, we peel them while keeping the tail on. We next use a knife to cut the shrimp's back to remove any black threads that may be inside. Put two prawns into each shell (or any other creative container you can think of) and then fill each one with a teaspoon of white wine so that the prawns are submerged in it. To make the panure, combine the breadcrumbs, salt, grated Parmigiano, and chopped parsley in a basin. Drizzle with oil and stir. Drizzle a little oil over the shells after covering them with a couple teaspoons of panure. Place the prawns and shells on a parchment paper-lined baking pan, and bake for approximately 25 minutes at 180 degrees. You are now prepared to present this creative cuisine!

Pineapple stuffed with shrimp

Ingredients:
- Pineapple of about 1 kg 1
- Shrimp 450 g
- Cherry tomatoes 240 g
- Chives 6 strands
- Mint 5 leaves
- Extra virgin olive oil to taste
- Salt to taste
- Mixed salad

Instructions

First, let's clean the prawns (you can also use frozen ones) by taking the fillet out of them. After giving them a quick wash under running water, use your hands to remove the legs and remove the head. Shell them now, please. After every prawn has been cleaned, coat a big pan with oil. Brown the peeled prawns on both sides after adding them to the pan. After that, turn off the heat and place them in a small basin to cool. Choose a ripe pineapple and cut it in half to prepare the pineapple that will hold your salad. Cut the inside pulp all the way around both halves so that you can remove all of the pulp without shattering it. Cut off the pulp's most callused area. Toss in the salad with medium-sized pineapple cubes made from the extracted pulp. Now slice the mint and chives for the aromas. The cherry tomatoes should then be cleaned under running water, drained, and chopped into small pieces.

After giving the mixed salad a quick rinse under the water, chop the pineapple and add the tomato pieces. Add the prawns that you previously sautéed. Next, add the chopped mint salt, chopped chives, and a drizzle of oil to the salad. Toss to combine the flavors. You can begin packing the pineapple until it is full now that the salad is done. You may now serve your salad with pineapple-topped shrimp for a lovely, light summer meal!

Chickpea shrimp and arugula salad

Ingredients:

- Shrimp 1 kg
- Pre-cooked chickpeas 240 g
- Rocket 150 g
- Pine nuts 30 g
- TO CONDITION
- Lemon juice 1
- Balsamic vinegar 1 tsp
- Extra virgin olive oil to taste
- Salt to taste

Instructions

The first step in preparing the chickpea shrimp and rocket salad is to clean the shrimp (or prawns) by taking out the head, carapace, and internal intestines.

Now, roast the pine nuts in a pan for four to five minutes, or until they turn brown.

Remove from the pan. Put the prawns in a skillet with some hot oil, salt, and a dash of pepper. Simmer them for five to six minutes on high heat. After they're done, move them to a small bowl to cool. After the pre cooked chickpeas have drained, you can use dried ones, but they must soak and cook for a minimum of three hours in order to be prepared. Heat the chickpeas in the same skillet as the prawns so they absorb the flavor of the seafood.

Now that everything is prepared, assemble the salad as follows: Place the washed and dry arugula in a large basin. Incorporate the prawns, chickpeas, and toasted pine nuts, blending thoroughly. Lastly, handle the dressing by making an emulsion with salt, oil, and half a lemon's juice.

Add a teaspoon of balsamic vinegar to finish. Apply the prepared dressing to the salad to season it. You can now prepare your rocket salad and chickpea shrimp.

Vegetable crudités

Ingredients:
- Celery 2
- Carrots 2
- Fennel 1
- Yellow peppers 1/2
- 1/2 red peppers
- Chicory 1
- Radishes 12
- Extra virgin olive oil to taste
- Lemon juice to taste
- Salt to taste

Instructions

Pick out two delicate celery stalks and trim off any leaves and filaments. After cutting the stalks into two equal-length sections, cut the sticks by chopping the portions that corresponded to the length. Remove the fennel's leafy ends first, and then the other one as well. Next, chop the fennel into four equal pieces, which you will then decrease in half once more. After removing the filaments and the white sections within the half peppers, cut the peppers into strips. After removing the radishes' leaves, give them a quick rinse under running water. After peeling and trimming the ends, cut the carrots into parallel slices, which you will later cut into sticks. Remove the radicchio's outer leaves, making sure to keep them apart from the plant's base so they stay fresh. Now arrange the chopped vegetables in tiny glasses and fill bowls with extra virgin olive oil. To prepare the sauce, mix together in a salt oil container, lemon, and beat vigorously with a fork to emulsify everything or do it with an immersion blender. Serve the sauce alongside your vegetable sticks.

Chunks of quinoa

Ingredients:
- Quinoa 150 g
- Small courgettes 2
- Eggs 1

- Grated cheese 50 g
- Grated lemon zest 1
- Fresh ginger to be grated to taste
- Salt to taste

Instructions

To stop the quinoa from cooking, drain it and rinse it in cold water. Peel and wash the courgettes at this step, and then peel and wash the fresh ginger. Grate the courgettes and transfer them to a big bowl. Add the grated lemon zest and fresh ginger to the bowl. When the courgettes, ginger, and lemon zest are shredded, add the boiled quinoa together with the grated cheese and egg. Add a pinch of salt and stir the ingredients until well combined. Now fill the molds with the mixture (you can alternatively use muffin tins that don't cling) and set them on a baking sheet. To properly define the shape of the morsels, compact the mixture inside the shapes using the back of a spoon.

Now, bake them for 25 minutes at 180 ° in static mode in an oven that has already been preheated (or 20 minutes at 160 ° in a fan oven) or until the tops are golden brown. The quinoa morsels are now prepared for consumption!

Eggplant Caviar

Ingredients:
- Round aubergines (about 3) 1 kg
- ½ lemon juice
- Mint 4 leaves
- Extra virgin olive oil 2 tbsp
- Salt to taste

Instructions

After giving the aubergines a wash under running water, pat dry. Place them in an arrangement on a parchment paper-lined drip pan. Bake them for at least 60 minutes at 180 ° in a preheated static oven (or for 50 minutes at 160 ° in a fan oven). Now take the aubergines out of the oven, cut off the peel with a knife, and scoop out the pulp using a spoon. Using the back of a spoon, press the pulp in a thin mesh strainer to release any remaining liquid. Place the pulp and oil into a mixer that has blades. After adding the mint and seasoning with salt, process the mixture with the blades until a thick, uniform puree is achieved.

After transferring everything to a small bowl, squeeze in the juice of half a lemon to create a puree.

Once everything is combined, your eggplant caviar is prepared for serving.

Octopus salad

Ingredients:

- Octopus to clean 1 kg
- Carrots 1
- Celery 1 rib
- Laurel 2 leaves
- Salt up to 4 g

TO CONDITION

- Parsley 10 g
- Lemon juice 10 g
- Extra virgin olive oil 30 g
- Black pepper 1 pinch
- Salt up to a pinch

Instructions

First, give the octopus a quick wash under running water. Next, remove the beak and use a knife to cut the bag around eye level. Rinse the octopus under running water once more, then carefully wash it inside the bag to remove the entrails (you can alternatively use the frozen one). After peeling, chop the carrot into rough pieces. Apply the same principle to celery. Put a large saucepan filled with water over medium heat, add the bay leaves, the chopped carrots, the chopped celery, and the salt. Once the water reaches a rolling boil, place the octopus in the pan and cook, covered, over very low heat for 40 to 45 minutes.

You can remove any residue or froth that forms on the water's surface while it cooks. Allow the octopus to chill in the same water after cooking until it becomes tender. After transferring it to the chopping board, split the tentacles in half and remove the head with a knife. Slice the tentacles into little segments. Chop the head into small pieces, then transfer all the contents into a bowl. Squeeze the lemon and wash and finely slice the parsley for the dressing. To make the dressing, combine the juice, oil, salt, parsley, and lemon juice in a jar. Mix and close. After thoroughly mixing and pouring the mixture over the octopus, serve your octopus salad!

Marinated anchovies

Ingredients:
- Anchovies (chopped) 500 g
- Lemon juice 150 g
- Parsley 20 g
- Extra virgin olive oil 140 g

- Fine salt

Instructions

In order to make the marinade for the marinated anchovies, combine the parsley and 40 grams of olive oil in a mixer and pulse to chop everything for a little while. After the lemons have been squeezed, put the juice, olive oil, and salt in a jar. Once the two compounds have combined thoroughly, stir in the chopped parsley. Stir continuously while setting aside the marinade. Proceed to clean the anchovies in the meantime. Since they won't be cooked, it's crucial to ensure that they were trimmed during the buying process (always choose fresh anchovies from a reputable fish store); for added safety, freeze the already-gutted anchovies for at least 96 hours at -18 degrees before thawing them out to use in the recipe. After removing the head, detach the middle bone and the entrails, and lastly give the fillets a thorough underwater rinsing, being cautious not to split the fish in half. After thoroughly cleaning the anchovy fillets, arrange them side by side in a big container, pour over the marinade, and cover with plastic wrap. Allow to stand at room temperature for a minimum of five hours.

Once the required amount of time has passed, take off the film, drain the anchovies gently from the marinade, and then arrange them on a platter to serve as an appetizer.

CHAPTER 3

FIRST DISHES

Risotto with chickpeas

Ingredients:
- 140 grams of brown rice
- 200 grams of boiled chickpeas
- 1 carrot
- 1 teaspoon of extra virgin olive oil
- vegetable broth

Add the oil to a skillet and sauté the small-cut carrots. 150 grams of cooked chickpeas should be combined and mixed to flavor everything. Cook the rice for a further fifteen minutes, or for as long as specified on the package.

If you notice that there is nothing liquid at the bottom of the pan, periodically add a ladle of vegetable rice broth. Add the leftover chickpeas to the cooked rice towards the end of cooking. It's time to enjoy your risotto!

Pasta and courgettes

Ingredients:
- Pasta 320 g
- Zucchini 650 g
- Basil to taste
- Salt to taste
- Extra virgin olive oil 20 g
- Black pepper to taste
- Garlic 1 clove

In a big pot, bring the water to a boil and add salt once it does. This will prepare the pasta and courgettes. Meanwhile, peel and pat dry the courgettes, then slice or cube them. Pour the extra virgin olive oil into a large enough pan and place a full peeled garlic clove inside. Heat the mixture over low heat. When the oil is hot, add the courgettes, season with salt and pepper, and cook, stirring periodically, for 5 to 6 minutes. After that, take out the garlic. Meanwhile, bring a pot of salted water to a boil, add the pasta, and cook it until it's al dente, setting aside some cooking water. Add the pasta to the pan with the zucchini and a small amount of cooking water. Stir and sauté the pasta for a few minutes before turning off. Once everything is fragrant, toss in some freshly chopped basil and serve your spaghetti and zucchini.

Legumes and cereals soup

Ingredients:

- Mixed legumes + cereals 500 g
- Carrots 2
- 2 ribs celery
- Onions 1
- Medium potatoes 2
- Auburn tomatoes 200 g
- Grana Padano DOP crusts 2
- Garlic 1 clove
- Vegetable broth 1 l

- Extra virgin olive oil 3 tbsp
- 1 sprig rosemary
- Thyme 1 sprig
- Bay leaf 1 leaf
- Sage 1 sprig

The day prior, soak the cereals in cold water. The next day, make sure they are fully drained before combining them with carrots, onion, garlic, and celery. In a large pot or crock, fry the mince in the oil. Add the drained grains and beans, stir for one minute, and then pour the vegetable broth over the top. Add the chopped and peeled tomatoes (into cubes). Add the grated Grana Padano crusts to the pan. At this point, add a bunch of aromatic herbs. Once cooked, you can quickly remove them by tying them to the pot's handle to prevent them from scattering throughout the soup.
Bring the soup to a gentle boil, add the salt, and then place a lid on the pan. Cook the soup slowly for at least an hour, adding

more vegetable broth as needed to keep the soup just the correct quantity of liquid. Add the diced and peeled potatoes 30 minutes before the food is done. Once cooked, remove the fragrant bunch and serve in bowls or holsters with a sprinkle of extra virgin olive oil.

Lentil soup

Ingredients:
- Lentils 250 g
- 2 ribs celery
- Carrots 2
- White onions 1
- Small potatoes 2
- 2 cloves garlic
- Zucchini 2
- Laurel 2 leaves
- Cumin 1 tsp
- Cloves 2
- Extra virgin olive oil 2 tbsp
- Salt to taste

- Boiling water 2,5 l

The day before, soak the lentils in cold water. Following the soaking period, begin cleaning the veggies. Peel and finely chop the carrots, celery (leaf removed), potatoes, and courgettes. In a skillet with high sides, heat the oil and add the garlic. Finely chop the onion and add it to the pan. Simmer the mixture for a little while before adding all the veggies, except the lentils. Cook over low heat, stirring occasionally, for about ten minutes. Once they are softened, add the lentils that have been well-drained from the soaking water, the bay leaves, the cloves, the cumin powder, and the salt. Finally, add the hot water, or vegetable broth, bring to a gentle boil, cover, and cook over low heat for about two hours, or until the lentils are well cooked and tender (but not falling apart). If the soup dries out too much, add more water.

Remove the bay leaves and maybe the cloves before putting it on the table, and serve it hot.

Quinoa with vegetables

Ingredients:
- Quinoa 200 g
- Champignon mushrooms 100 g
- Red peppers 70 g
- Yellow peppers 70 g
- Courgettes 150 g
- Red onions 100 g
- Water 400 g
- Extra virgin olive oil to taste
- Mint to taste
- Salt to taste
- Black pepper to taste

First, wash and finely chop the red onions before preparing the quinoa with veggies. Remove the seeds from inside the red pepper by cutting it in half. After that, chop it into cubes and proceed the same way with the yellow pepper. Next, clean and slice the mushrooms after chopping the courgettes into cubes. Add the onions to a pan with hot oil. Allow them to cook slowly for a few minutes until they are extremely soft. When they start to brown, mix them with a little water. When this is finished, add the peppers, stir, and simmer for a few more minutes before adding the mushrooms and zucchini. Add salt and pepper and cook for an additional five minutes. Your veggies are prepared and gorgeously crunchy! Now handle the quinoa: rinse it well, then add it to a skillet with hot oil on the bottom to toast it. Add the salt and stir with a wooden spoon to make sure it doesn't stick to the bottom. Cook the remaining water, making sure that its volume is double that of the quinoa, and cover. The quinoa is done when the seeds open to flower and the water is absorbed; at that time, you can mix them with the vegetables. Add with a handful of mint leaves after mixing and pausing for a minute to meld the flavors. It's time to enjoy quinoa with vegetables!

Spaghetti with tuna

Ingredients:
- Spaghetti 320 g
- Tuna in oil (drained) 150 g
- Peeled tomatoes 400 g
- Extra virgin olive oil to taste
- Salt to taste
- Black pepper to taste
- Basil to taste
- Golden onions ½

In order to make the spaghetti with tuna, first bring a kettle of water to a boil, add salt, and cook the pasta. Empty the tuna fillet's conservation oil in the interim. After cleaning, thinly slice the onion. Add chopped onion to a skillet with olive oil. Stirring often, let it dry on the stove for a few minutes.

When the onion has dried, remove the tuna with your hands, add it to the pan, and stir continuously while allowing it to brown for a few minutes. Now, add the peeled tomatoes to the pan with the tuna and use a fork to mash them. Cook the sauce for ten minutes or so. The pasta will be ready during the seasoning's cooking period. After draining and adding fresh basil leaves to the pan with the tuna, season with ground pepper and turn off the heat. Serve your hot pasta with tuna after stirring!

Chickpea and pumpkin soup

Ingredients:
- Delica pumpkin to clean 600 g
- Drained pre-cooked chickpeas 400 g
- Beets 100 g
- Golden onions 100 g
- Juniper berries 3 berries
- Laurel 2 leaves

- Water 1.5 l
- Extra virgin olive oil to taste
- Salt to taste
- Black pepper to taste

First, wash the onion and thinly slice it before making the chickpea and pumpkin soup. You will need 430 g of clean pumpkin after cleaning it by cutting it in half, taking out the seeds, and removing the peel. Dice the pulp with a knife. After washing, thinly slice the beets. Add the juniper berries and the sliced onion to a skillet with olive oil. Allow the onion to simmer on low heat until it becomes tender. Add the pumpkin at this point, brown it over medium heat, and then moisten it with a small amount of water from the entire dosage. Add the chickpeas, the chard that has been reduced to 11 strips, salt, pepper, and the remaining boiling water.

Add bay leaves for flavor, stir, put a lid on, and simmer over high heat for fifteen minutes.

Take off the lid and cook for a further fifteen minutes. After taking out the juniper berries and bay leaves, serve your soup with minced black pepper and a drizzle of raw oil. The soup made with pumpkin and chickpeas is prepared for serving.

Pasta with eggplants

Ingredients:
- Striped Sedanini 320 g
- Aubergines 350 g
- Cherry tomatoes 250 g
- Basil a few leaves
- Fresh spring onion 100 g
- Salt to taste
- Black pepper to taste
- Extra virgin olive oil 30 g

After washing and chopping the aubergines, cook the pasta with them. After that, move them to a colander, sprinkle them liberally with salt, cover them with a saucer that is weighted, and allow them to drain for a few hours. Slice the spring onion thinly after the aubergines have completely released their water. Once the oil has warmed up, add the spring onion to the pan. After it turns golden brown, simmer for approximately 15 minutes after adding the aubergines and salt and pepper. After washing, cut the tomatoes into wedges, and add them to the aubergines just after they have cooked through and soft. After adding salt and pepper, simmer for an additional four to five minutes.

Meanwhile, cook the pasta in plenty of salted boiling water. After it's cooked through, drain it and transfer it straight into the pan with the aubergines. Add the basil leaves 1 instead of pasta with aubergines; all you need to do now is serve.

Vegetable pie

Ingredients:
- Aubergines 80 g
- Zucchini 160 g
- Red potatoes 190 g
- Peppers 300 g
- Smoked scamorza 260 g
- PDO Parmesan Cheese 100 g
- Breadcrumbs 120 g
- Salt to taste
- Extra virgin olive oil to taste

FOR THE TRAY
- Butter to taste
- Breadcrumbs to taste

Wash and dry all the vegetables before beginning to make the vegetable pie.

Prepare the aubergines by peeling, slicing them in half, and then cutting them into slices that are approximately 1 cm thick (a mandolin can come in handy for this). Repeat with the courgettes, and lastly cut the potatoes into slices without peeling them. Now take the peppers, cut off the tops, split them in half, and then take out the seeds and stems. Lastly, split into six halves.

Lastly, cut the scamorza into pieces the same thickness as the veggies. Line the bottom of a baking dish with grease and breadcrumbs. Proceed to creating the layers at this point. Place all of the aubergine slices on the base to begin. Add a little parmesan, breadcrumbs, and a few slices of scamorza cheese after sprinkling with oil and salt. Next, arrange the zucchini slices, season with oil and salt, and then scatter the breadcrumbs, scamorza, and parmesan cheese over them. Lastly, using peppers once again. Repeat with the final layer, the potato layer, and season with salt, oil, parmesan, and breadcrumbs. Finally, top the last layer with breadcrumbs, salt, and parmesan cheese. Sprinkle with oil.

Next, continue cooking for around 70 minutes and 20 minutes in a static oven that has been warmed to 180 degrees. When ready, let it cool. Move to a platter for serving.

Rice cake

Ingredients:
- Champignon mushrooms 500 g
- Rice 300 g
- Grated cheese 150 g
- ½ white onions
- Vegetable broth about 750 ml
- White wine 60 ml
- Parsley 1 sprig
- Salt to taste

Start by cleaning and chopping the onion in order to prepare the rice cake. Next, commit yourself to the champignon mushrooms. Give them a thorough cleaning and washing. Next, cut the tops of the mushrooms into thin slices and remove the portion of the stem that contains the roots. Slice the new parsley. Drizzle some oil in a big pan and add the chopped parsley and champignon mushrooms. After about three minutes of low heat cooking, add thirty milliliters of white wine. For roughly five minutes, stir and cook the mushrooms. Add salt for seasoning, then simmer over medium heat for approximately ten minutes. The mushrooms will finish cooking in the oven, so they won't need to cook all the way through. As the mushrooms cook, add the chopped onion to a big skillet with oil and saute it for around five minutes. After that, add the rice, mix it with a wooden spoon for a few minutes while it sautes, and then add the last milliliter of white wine.

Once the rice is completely dry, continue cooking the risotto for another 20 minutes or more, gradually adding the vegetable stock with a ladle.

Add the grated cheese, mix, and turn off the heat when the rice has two minutes remaining in its cooking time. Allow the risotto to rest for a few minutes. First, line a baking sheet with parchment paper. Next, begin layering the rice with a spoon, pressing it down with the back of the spoon. After covering the bottom, add a layer of rice and mushrooms together to make two layers with the mushroom filling. Lastly, scatter the remaining cheese over the surface. Lastly, bake for about 30 minutes at 200 ° in a static oven that has been prepared (or for about 25 minutes at 180 °). After that, remove it from the oven and allow it to cool.

CHAPTER 4

MAIN COURSES

Veal roast, apples and potatoes

Ingredients:
- 600 grams of veal fillet
- 1 teaspoon of oil
- 2 sprigs of rosemary
- half a glass of white wine
- 2 apples
- 250 grams of potatoes
- Salt

Place the meat in a pan with a little oil, salt, and rosemary. Blend it with the white wine to get a brown color. Add the cut potatoes and the apples with the peel. Bake for about thirty minutes at 200 degrees. Take the meat out of the oven and allow it to cool. Slice it and serve it with apples and potatoes.

Poached eggs

Ingredients:

- Very fresh, organic eggs 4
- Coarse salt to taste
- White wine vinegar 10 g
- TO ACCOMPANY
- 4 slices bread

Once the salt has dissolved and the water begins to gently boil (it shouldn't boil violently), turn down the heat and whisk continuously in the same direction to agitate the water and produce a vortex. Crack an egg into a small dish and place it in the center of the vortex. This way, cook the egg for two minutes.

Never stir or agitate the egg. Using a slotted spoon to drain the egg, place it over the toast and serve your hot poached eggs.

Prawns stewed

Ingredients:

- King prawns (12 pieces) 600 g
- Peeled tomatoes (cherry tomatoes) 400 g
- Water 200 g
- Brandy 50 g
- Extra virgin olive oil 30 g
- Garlic 1 clove
- Parsley to taste
- Salt to taste

To prepare the prawns for stewing, begin by carefully cleaning them by removing the outermost layer of carapace and the dark filament by drawing it out with a toothpick or knife. Arrange the prawns on a tray, leaving the head and tail connected. Add a whole peeled garlic clove to a skillet of heated olive oil. Once the oil is heated, arrange the prawns in a pan so that they are not overlapping and brown on both sides for one minute. Next, mix in the brandy and add the peeled cherry tomatoes, allowing the sauce to thicken with water. Add the salt, place the lid on, and simmer for an additional five minutes or so. Using kitchen tongs, remove the garlic clove. Next, crush some of the cherry tomatoes with a fork. Cook the prawns for a further 10 minutes or so. Clean, pat dry, and roughly slice the parsley.

Once done, remove from the heat and toss the prawns with freshly chopped parsley before serving hot from the skillet.

Sea bass with herb in salt crust

Ingredients:
- Salt up to 1 kg
- Sea bass (sea bass) 800 g
- Coarse salt 1 kg
- Sage 6 leaves
- Thyme 6 sprigs
- Parsley 1 bunch
- Dill 2 tufts

- Laurel 4 leaves
- Rosemary 3 sprigs
- Egg whites about 4
- Garlic 1 clove
- Lemons 1

Chicken and courgette salad

Ingredients:
- Sliced chicken breast 400 g
- Zucchini 200 g
- Eggplants 200 g
- Datterini tomatoes 150 g
- Mixed salad 60 g
- Salt to taste
- Extra virgin olive oil to taste

FOR MARINATING
- Extra virgin olive oil 25 g
- Wildflower honey 25 g
- ½ lemon juice
- Thyme to taste
- Salt to taste

We need to marinade the chicken first before making the chicken and courgette salad. Place the chicken breasts in an ovenproof dish, cover with oil, and season with salt, honey, lemon juice, and a few thyme sprigs. After flipping the slices over to ensure that the meat is fully marinated on all sides, cover the baking dish with plastic wrap and leave it to rest at room temperature for an hour. Proceed to the veggie preparation now. After washing, trim the ends of the courgettes and cut them lengthwise with a slicing knife that is approximately 1 cm thick. Apply the same method to eggplants as well.

Lastly, give the cherry tomatoes a quick wash and chop. Now preheat the grill, coat it with a thin layer of oil, place the zucchini slices there, grill on both sides, and season with salt. Furthermore, cook and salt the aubergines, flipping them over on both sides. Next, go on to the chicken, which you will remove from the marinade and grill.

After grilling, cut the chicken slices, courgettes, and aubergines into strips that are roughly 2 cm long. After allowing the grilled veggies to cool, move them to a bowl, stir in the cherry tomatoes, chicken, and mixed salad (which has already been cleaned and dried), and then serve. It's time to serve the zucchini and chicken salad!

Pan-fried sea bream

Ingredients:
- Sea bream (2 pieces) 1100 g
- Extra virgin olive oil 30 g
- Carrots 150 g
- Courgettes 150 g
- Fresh spring onion 70 g
- Garlic 1 clove
- Thyme to taste

Cleaning the fish is the first step in preparing sea bream in a pan (you can purchase it already gutted). Using scissors, cut a hole in the abdomen and remove the entrails with your hands. Rinse the interior well with water and use a knife blade to remove the scales; do this under running water to prevent the scales from spreading. The vegetables need to be cut now. First, wash and peel the carrots. Then, trim the ends and cut the carrots into rounds. Cut the courgettes into cubes after washing and peeling them. Lastly, give the onion a wash, take off the base, and slice it into rounds. A clove of poached garlic should be added to a big nonstick pan filled with oil, and it should be cooked for a few minutes. After the oil has taken on flavor, take out the garlic and place the sea bream within the pan. Next, add the carrots, zucchini, spring onions, thyme sprigs, and salt to taste.

After cooking the sea bream for seven minutes on medium heat with a lid on, flip them over using two spatulas, being cautious not to smash them, and cook for a further seven minutes with the lid still on.

Depending on the weight of the sea bream you use, cooking times may change.
Sea bream cooked in a pan is ready to eat!

Cod medallions and broccoli

Ingredients:
- Cod fillet 400 g
- Broccoli 200 g
- Potatoes 400 g
- Marjoram 3 sprigs
- Extra virgin olive oil to taste
- Salt to taste

TO ACCOMPANY
- Cherry tomatoes 200 g
- Dried oregano to taste
- Extra virgin olive oil to taste
- Salt to taste

First, we take the cod fillets (which should ideally be frozen; if not, let them defrost for at least two to three hours beforehand) and prepare them for the cod and broccoli medallions. After that, place two saucepans over medium heat and fill them with water to the boil. Cook the potatoes for 30 to 40 minutes in one of the saucepans. Remember to use a fork to verify the potatoes' level of doneness as cooking times can vary according on their size. When a fork readily pierces through potatoes, it indicates that they are cooked. Wash the broccoli, transfer it to the other pan, and cook it for around five minutes once the water reaches a boil. The broccoli should be drained after five minutes, roughly chopped, and allowed to cool. When the potatoes are ready, put them in a big bowl, peel and mash with a potato masher, and then turn the oven on to 200° in static mode. Lastly, remove the cod fillets and chop them into a few little pieces.

After the vegetables have cooled, take the bowl with the mashed potatoes and add the chopped cod and broccoli. Season with salt and add the marjoram leaves. Using your hands, knead the items together. Using a pastry cutter, mold some dough into the desired shape for the medallions. After seasoning with a little oil and placing the medallions on a parchment paper-lined dripping pan, preheat a static oven to 200 °C for around 20 minutes.

While the medallions are in the oven, prepare the side dish by washing and halving the cherry tomatoes. Then, add the salt and oregano to the pan with the cherry tomatoes and cook over medium heat for approximately 15 minutes. Once the medallions have finished cooking, remove them from the oven and place them on a platter. Arrange the tomatoes, which are still hot, on one side and sprinkle with some marjoram leaves and raw oil. The medallions of fish and broccoli are prepared for serving!

Baked chicken legs

Ingredients:

- Chicken legs 4
- Potatoes 500 g
- Salt to taste
- Extra virgin olive oil 50 g
- Rosemary 3 sprigs
- Thyme 3 sprigs

Season the chicken legs with salt, oil, and marinade before placing them in a baking dish.

After peeling and cutting the potatoes into wedges, place them in a parchment paper-lined drip pan. Season everything with salt, oil, and pepper (don't overdo it), then add the chicken legs and the rosemary and thyme sprigs. Preheat a static oven to 180 °C and bake for 80 minutes, rotating them halfway through. Remove from the oven and serve after they are golden brown!

Stuffed potatoes
Ingredients:
- Potatoes (4 of the same size) 860 g

- Ground beef 120 g
- Sweet provola 40 g
- Grated Parmesan cheese 40 g
- Extra virgin olive oil 30 g
- White wine 15 g
- Salt to taste

Wash and pat dry the potatoes thoroughly before beginning to cook the baked filled potatoes. Selecting potatoes with similar sizes can help ensure consistent cooking in the end. Place the potatoes in an arrangement on a parchment paper-covered drip pan. For approximately one hour, cook them in a static oven that has been prepared to 190°C. The amount of time needed to cook depends on the size of the potatoes; use a toothpick to test them to see how they are done. Meanwhile, add the minced beef to a skillet of heated oil.

Once the alcohol has disappeared, blend it with white wine, crush it until crumbly, and brown it for approximately ten minutes.

Then, turn off the heat and set aside. After the potatoes are done cooking, remove from the oven, allow to cool, and then cut in half lengthwise. Using a teaspoon, remove the potato pulp, leaving a half-cm border around it, and transfer it to a bowl. After the potatoes have been removed, purée the pulp and add the seasoned and browned mince. Provola should be cut into cubes and added to the recipe, thoroughly mixing the ingredients. Now stuff the filling into your potatoes. After seasoning the potatoes with the grated cheese, place them on a parchment paper-covered dripping pan and bake for five minutes at 180 °C to brown the top. Warm up your filled baked potatoes.

Roasted rabbit

Ingredients:
- Rabbit in pieces 1.2 kg
- 4 sprigs rosemary
- Salt to taste

- Vegetable broth 150 g
- Potatoes 800 g
- Red onions 120 g
- Thyme 4 sprigs
- White wine 40 g
- Bay leaf 1 leaf
- Extra virgin olive oil 70 g

In order to prepare the rabbit for baking, begin by making the vegetable broth a few hours in advance. Chop the rosemary and then put half of it into a skillet with 40 grams of oil in it. After adding a bay leaf, cook for two to three minutes on low heat to flavor it. Now turn up the heat and add the rabbit pieces. Cook for three to four minutes on each side, then season with salt and stir in the white wine. After the alcohol has evaporated, simmer for a further five to six minutes over low heat while adding a ladle of broth. In the meantime, prepare the potatoes by peeling and chopping them into sizable chunks. Additionally, chop the onion and add it to a bowl along with the salt and chopped rosemary that you set aside before. To flavor the potatoes, combine them with onions and sprinkle with 20 g of oil. Place everything in a big pan that has been lightly greased with 10 g of oil. Next, place the browned rabbit pieces as well. After adding the remaining vegetable broth, boil the rabbit and potatoes for 40 minutes at 200° in a static oven that has been warmed. Serve your cooked rabbit straight from the oven!

CHAPTER 5

RECIPES FOR SIDE DISH

Fennel in a pan

Ingredients:

- Fennel (about 2) 900 g
- Extra virgin olive oil 15 g
- Himalayan salt (pink) to taste
- Marjoram to taste
- Thyme to taste

In order to prepare fennel for frying, first wash the leaves, then trim the ends and base of the stalks, chopping them into wedges. After chopping the fennel, you can start cooking it by heating some extra virgin olive oil in a pan, adding the sliced fennel, and cooking it on high for about five minutes. Season with the Himalayan salt and the thyme and marjoram leaves. If you prefer softer fennel, you can simmer them for a few more minutes. If not, roast them for a further five minutes to keep them crunchy. In a pan, serve your fennel hot.

Baked aubergines

Ingredients:
- 2 cloves garlic
- Extra virgin olive oil to taste
- Salt to taste
- Aubergines 970 g
- Auburn tomatoes 500 g
- Chopped parsley 3 tbsp

You can use both the rotunda and the elongated violet variety of aubergine to make baked aubergine. Slices of aubergine should first be cleaned.

After salting, put the aubergine slices in a colander. To compress them, cover them with a plate that will hold weight, and let them sit for 30 minutes to allow the bitter liquid to evaporate. In the meantime, wash the tomatoes, cut them in half, and carefully scrape out the seeds using a little knife inside. Cut them into little pieces now, and transfer them to a bowl. Add the salt, oil, and three spoons of finely chopped parsley to the tomatoes to season them now. After mixing, let the tomato chunks macerate in the dressing for a short while. After 30 minutes, pick up the eggplant slices and make sure the bitter water has been expelled. After giving them a quick rinse in cold running water, pat them dry with a kitchen towel or cloth. Preheat the static oven to 180–200 degrees.

Apply olive oil to a baking pan with high sides and begin layering aubergines.

Next, add a layer of cherry tomatoes on top. This process should be repeated until all the aubergines have been used. Next, bake the dish for at least 40 minutes at 200° in a static oven that has been preheated. Eating is possible both hot and cold.

Grilled vegetables

Ingredients:

- Courgettes 300 g
- Eggplants 450 g
- Peppers 850 g
- Tomatoes 200 g
- Salt to taste

Clean all the veggies under running water and pat dry before preparing the grilled veggies. Slice the aubergines and courgettes; take the peppers, cut off the tops, then cut them in half, removing the seeds and white filaments inside with a knife. Chop them into fairly large cubes and reserve. Cut the tomatoes into rounds after removing the stalks. Assemble all the veggies and preheat the grill. Cook the vegetables a little at a time once the grill is hot. Arrange the peppers closely together and grill for 5 minutes, flipping them over to ensure equal cooking. After 3 minutes, place the eggplants and courgettes over the fire, and continue cooking for an additional 3 minutes.

Always remember to flip the veggies to ensure they cook evenly. Cook the tomatoes for a further 4 minutes, or until they are nicely grilled. Finally, add salt and olive oil to the grilled veggies.

Mashed potatoes

Ingredients:
- Yellow floury potatoes 1 kg
- Whole milk 200 g
- Butter 30 g
- Parmesan cheese to be grated 30 g
- Salt to taste
- Nutmeg to taste

First, let's boil the potatoes. After that, transfer them into a big pot and add lots of water to cover. It will take 40 to 50 minutes for the water to boil after you put the pan on the stove. The size of the potatoes affects how long they need to cook. When the 40 minutes have passed, test the doneness of the potato by skewering it with a fork to check if it easily penetrates; if so, it is done. Drain and allow to cool for a few minutes, as you will need to take advantage of the potatoes' extreme heat to facilitate easy peeling. Once the potatoes have been peeled, transfer them straight into the cooking pan using the potato masher. Next, season with a pinch of salt and a small grating of nutmeg. Meanwhile, transfer the milk to a saucepan.

In the meantime, place a pot with mashed potatoes over a low heat. Once the milk is ready, pour it inside and stir to thoroughly combine the ingredients. After that, turn off the heat and whisk in the Parmesan cheese and butter. It reads "mashed potato" for you.

Baked au gratin vegetables

Ingredients:

- Courgettes 300 g

- Aubergines 180 g long
- Red peppers 250 g
- Yellow peppers 250 g
- Extra virgin olive oil 20 g
- Salt to taste

FOR BREADING

- Breadcrumbs 30 g
- Parmesan cheese DOP to be grated 30 g
- Dried oregano to taste

Cut the veggies first. Wash the aubergines, trim the ends, and cut them into 2-3 cm thick slices on the diagonal. Repeat with the zucchini. Lastly, wash the peppers, remove the seeds and internal filaments, and cut them into pieces that are roughly the same size as the slices of zucchini and aubergine. After chopping the vegetables, place them in a parchment paper-lined skillet and toss with olive oil and salt. Bake the pan for 45 minutes at 180° in a static oven that has been prepared. Meanwhile, get the breadcrumbs ready for the veggies:

Combine the breadcrumbs, oregano, and grated Parmesan cheese in a bowl and well combine. After the vegetables have been cooking for 45 minutes, take them out of the oven and use a spoon to coat each one in breadcrumbs. Bake for a further fifteen minutes at 180 °. It's time for your side dish!

Artichoke salad

Ingredients:
- Artichokes (about 6) 1 kg
- Lemons for acidulated water 1

FOR THE CITRONETTE
- Lemon juice 30 g
- Salt to taste
- Black pepper to taste
- Extra virgin olive oil 60

To begin, wash the artichokes and set aside enough acidulated water to keep them fresh while you clean them. Pour some water into a bowl and add one lemon's juice. Take off the more leathery leaves and a portion of the artichokes' stem. To keep the inside of the stem soft, trim off the tip and the outermost portion with a knife.

After cleaning and dividing it into two equal halves, thinly slice the artichokes and drop them, cut-side down, into the bowl of water that has been acidified.

After cleaning is complete, place them in a colander to drain. Attend the seasoning in the meanwhile. 30 grams of freshly squeezed lemon juice, 60 grams of olive oil, salt, and whisked emulsion are combined. After adding the citronette to the bowl of artichokes, stir, and arrange the salad on the serving dishes!

Breadcrumb Potatoes

Ingredients:
- Potatoes 1 kg
- 2 sprigs rosemary
- Bread crumbs 50 g

- Breadcrumbs 20 g
- Sage 3 leaves
- Extra virgin olive oil to taste
- Salt to taste

To prevent them from becoming black, peel and chop the potatoes into wedges. Then, put them in a bowl of water. Meanwhile, chop the rosemary and sage finely and set them aside. Add the breadcrumbs and the chopped herbs to the breadcrumbs now. Now use a strainer to remove the potato wedges, then add the breadcrumbs and season with salt and olive oil.

After giving them a stir, transfer the potatoes onto a baking dish covered with parchment paper. Then, sprinkle some bread crumbs over them. In a static oven, bake the potatoes for 40 minutes at 180 °C (or 30 minutes at 160 °C). Your potatoes should be crispy and golden when done; remove from the oven and allow to cool before serving.

Crunchy salad

Ingredients:
- Iceberg salad 1 large head
- PDO Parmigiano Reggiano one piece or in flakes 80 g
- Carrots 2
- 4 slices sandwich bread
- Chopped parsley 3 tbsp
- Anchovies fillets 8
- Lemon juice
- Salt to taste
- Extra virgin olive oil 2 tablespoons for frying, plus q.s. to season

After washing and finely chopping, place the iceberg salad leaves in a big salad dish. Now pass the carrots and use a potato peeler to chop them finely. Repeat with the Parmesan cheese, using the potato peeler throughout. Chop the parsley and anchovy fillets, then put them in a bowl with oil and salt. Using a fork, mix everything together, and let it sit for a few minutes.

After removing the darker corners from the sandwich bread pieces, cut each slice into a cube that is one centimeter on each side. Two teaspoons of extra virgin olive oil should be added to a skillet, warmed, and then tossed with the bread cubes over a medium heat, turning them over on all sides. When golden, transfer them to a piece of absorbent kitchen paper 11. To the iceberg salad, add the carrots, Parmesan, oil, and parsley dressing. After combining the ingredients, stir in the crunchy croutons 15. Salad prepared ahead of time!

Ginger gourd

Ingredients:
- Pumpkin 1 kg
- Fresh ginger 40 g
- Leeks 1
- Vegetable broth 500 ml
- Extra virgin olive oil 20 g
- Salt to taste

Cleaning the pumpkin, cutting it in half, removing the peel, and chopping it into cubes should be our first steps. then chop it into tiny cubes. Peel and wash the leek, saving the white portion of the stem to cut into thin slices. Set a large pan over medium heat, add the leeks, season with the olive oil, and cook for about 5 minutes, or until the leeks wilt.

At this stage, add the ginger, pumpkin cubes, and salt to a ladle of heated soup.

Pour in another ladle of liquid and simmer for 25 to 30 minutes on medium heat, adding broth little by little so as not to overcook the veggies. Switch off the heat once the pumpkin is tender. It's time to set the ginger pumpkin on the table.

Roasted carrots with pistachio

Ingredients:

- Carrots 650 g
- Unsalted pistachios 80 g

- Rosemary 3 sprigs
- Salt to taste
- Extra virgin olive oil to taste

After giving the carrots a wash and peeling them, cut them into long sticks by slicing them in half. Transfer the carrots into a bowl and add salt, olive oil, and rosemary for seasoning. Now use a knife to roughly chop the pistachios. Toss to combine all the ingredients, then add the pistachios and carrots. To make cooking easier, line a baking sheet with parchment paper and add the carrots, spreading them out evenly. Bake for 30 minutes at 220 ° in a static oven that has been prepared. Before serving, remove the cooked roasted carrots from the oven and allow them to cool.

CHAPTER 6

RECIPES FOR DESSERT

Cake Seven Jars

Ingredients:

- Natural white yogurt (125 ml) at room temperature 1 jar
- Brown sugar 2 jars
- flour 2 jars
- Potato starch 1 jar
- Seed oil 1 jar
- Baking powder for sweets 16 g
- Medium eggs at room temperature 3

To make the seven jar cake, take a 125 ml jar of room-temperature whole yogurt and put it in a basin. Next, add two jars of sugar and begin whisking the mixture until it becomes a smooth cream. Now crack the eggs and divide the yolks and whites into two different bowls. Add the yolks to the yogurt and sugar mixture and beat until combined, using the mixer once more. Continue to add the oil equally while the mixer is running. After everything is thoroughly combined, put a sieve right on top of the bowl and add the two jars of flour, the starch jar, and then the baking powder sachet.

Everything should be sieved, and the powders should always be added while using the low-speed mixer to create a smooth, homogenous mixture. Now take the egg whites and beat them until they form firm peaks. Add them two or three times to your mixture: To prevent the compound from disintegrating, add a little amount of egg whites at first and beat quickly without worrying about inflating the dough. Next, add the remaining egg whites and beat softly while rotating the mixture from the bottom up. When the cake dough is finished, flour and butter a 24 cm round mold, and then fill it with the batter. Now bake the seven jars of cake in a static oven that has been warmed to 180 ° for 45 minutes; during the final 10 minutes of baking, cover the cake with aluminum foil if it starts to become black on top. Test with a toothpick to make sure it's cooked through, then remove from the oven and allow to cool before slicing and serving.

Chiffon Cake

Ingredients:
- Sugar 300 g
- flour 290 g
- Water 200 g
- Sunflower oil 120 g
- Large eggs 6
- Vanilla bean 1
- Untreated lemon zest 1
- Sweet baking powder 1 sachet
- Salt up to 2 g
- Icing sugar to taste

In order to make the chiffon cake, begin by sifting the flour and yeast in a bowl. Add the salt and sugar after that. Stir to ensure optimal mixing. Six large eggs should have their yolks separated from their whites in a different bowl. The egg whites should be left aside. To the yolks, add the seed oil and room-temperature water. Next, finely grate the lemon rind, cut open a vanilla bean, remove the seeds, and include them into the yolk mixture. Using a whisk, beat the mixture until it becomes uniform. Next, pour it all at once into the dry ingredients (yeast, sugar, and flour). Using a whisk, thoroughly stir until creamy. Give this dough some time to rest, and then set aside some time to beat the egg whites.

Once the egg whites are frothy, pour them into the bowl of a planetary mixer (you may use an electric mixer if you don't have one). Turn on the whisk and begin whisking the egg whites. After the egg whites are thoroughly beaten, scoop some of the mixture into the reserved dough and immediately stir with a spatula to thin it out. Next, gradually add the remaining egg whites, mixing constantly from top to bottom with a spatula.

When the cake dough is done, carefully pour it into the chiffon cake mold, which measures 10 cm high, 26 cm on the top, and 22 cm in the bottom. Make an effort to divide the dough equally. Next, bake the chiffon cake for approximately 60 minutes in a 160 ° static oven (or 45−50 minutes in a 150 ° ventilated oven), with the cake placed in the lowest third of the oven.

After cooking, remove from the oven and let it cool. Using a small, sharp knife, you can assist yourself by removing the upper portion of the mold once the chiffon cake has completely cooled. You can now freely dust your chiffon cake with powdered sugar!

Stuffed peaches in the oven

Ingredients:

- Medium, ripe and firm yellow peaches 800 g
- Dark chocolate 100 g
- Amaretti 80 g

Rinse and rinse the peaches first before preparing the stuffed ones for the oven. Using a tiny knife, cut each peach in half to remove the core.

Additionally, remove some pulp from around the core's hollow while setting the peaches aside. Now set yourself to work on the filling: slice the peach pulp and set it aside. Chop up the chocolate finely and set it aside. Take another bowl and coarsely crumble the macaroons inside. If you'd like, you may also use a mixer to chop them finely. To the crumbled amaretti, add the peach pulp. Combine the ingredients, then stir in the chocolate. Spoon a little bit of the filling into each peach so that it forms a tiny dome. Lastly, arrange the peaches closely together in a baking dish that has been lightly greased, ideally leaving no gaps. Bake for 60 minutes at 180 °C in a static preheated oven (or for 50 minutes in a fan oven at 160 °C). When the allotted amount of time has passed, remove the filled peaches and serve them to your guests hot!

Sweet made soon

Ingredients:
- Sugar 200 g
- flour 220 g
- Butter 150 g
- Medium eggs 4
- Untreated lemon zest 1
- Vanilla bean 1
- Baking powder 8 g

In a planetary mixer fitted with whips, begin by adding the sugar and the softened butter and stirring the mixture. After that, chop a stick of vanilla and add the seeds to the concoction. After grating the zest from the lemon, beat the room temperature eggs. Once the mixture is completely combined, stop the mixer and sift the flour and yeast into a bowl. Add the bowl to the mixture and stir everything together thoroughly. Pour the mixture into a donut mold that has been floured and greased. To disperse it equally, use a spatula to spread it. The cake can be baked for 50 minutes at 170° in a prepared static oven or for around 40 minutes at 150° in a vented oven. Make sure the cake is done by inserting a toothpick into it before baking. The cake is done when a toothpick inserted into it comes out clean. Allow the cake to cool completely before completing the recipe by dusting it with powdered sugar.

Fruit ice cream

Ingredients:
- Melon 1.2 kg

- Pineapple 2 kg
- Mango 600 g
- Strawberries 500 g
- Blackberries 500 g

Cleanse the melon first. Segment the melon in half after cutting off the ends.

Take out the seeds; cut each half into thin slices; take off the peel from each slice; and then chop them into cubes that are about 2 cm thick. Place the cubes in a tray, taking care not to stack them on top of one another, wrap in plastic wrap, and place in the freezer. Once the fruit has solidified, it can be placed in a frost bag and left for a minimum of twelve hours. Proceed to clean the pineapple by cutting off the tuft and base, dividing it into four sections, removing the wooden core, and finally removing the peel.

Each segment should be cut in half, and the resulting slices should be roughly 1 cm thick. Next, arrange the pineapple on a tray, cover it with plastic wrap, and place it in the freezer. Once the pineapple has solidified, it should always be placed in a bag and left to freeze for at least 12 hours.

Cleaning the mango involves removing the peel, cutting each slice individually with a knife for a considerable amount of time until the core is still in your hand; then, cut each slice into cubes that are about 2 cm thick, spread evenly on a tray, cover with plastic wrap, and freeze for at least 12 hours. The strawberries need to be taken care of now. First, wash and dry them. Next, cut them in half and remove the stalk. At this point, place the strawberries on a tray without overlapping and freeze for at least 12 hours. Lastly, give the blackberries a gentle wash and dry before putting them whole on a tray and freezing for a minimum of 12 hours. Once the fruit has frozen, you can blend it to make a cool dessert. Simply place the frozen melon in a bowl or blender with steel blades and process until it turns creamy.

Similarly, add the frozen pineapple, strawberries, and frozen blackberries to the blender and process until the mixture has a creamy consistency. Serve your frozen fruit right away by transferring it into different bowls!

Sweet beetroot cake

Ingredients:
- Sugar 190 g
- flour 260 g
- Pre-cooked beets 400 g
- Dark chocolate 130 g
- Corn seed oil 230 g
- Eggs 3
- Baking powder for sweets 16 g
- Van pod

First, we peel and cube the beets that have previously been cooked. After that, move them to the immersion mixer's glass, stretch them with a trickle of oil (about 30 g total;

this is required for the recipe), and blend. Set aside the beet cream and proceed with the chocolate by roughly chopping it and letting it dissolve in a water bath. Once it has melted entirely, set it aside to cool.

Until then, commit yourself to the dough. Pour the room-temperature eggs and sugar into the mixer (you can also use an electric mixer), add the vanilla bean seeds, and run the whisk. Work the mixture into a thick froth before adding the oil and continuing to work. Gradually incorporate the flour and baking powder into the dough after sieving them. To ensure a flawless mixing, add the cold chocolate last and keep kneading the dough for a few more minutes. Using a spatula, carefully whisk the beetroot cream into the dough until it is well absorbed.

Next, transfer the dough into a cake tin with a 24 cm diameter that has been coated with parchment paper and buttered beforehand. Before baking, insert a toothpick to check for doneness. Bake in a preheated static oven for 65 minutes at 170 degrees (or 55 minutes if the oven is ventilated). Take the cake out of the oven and allow it to cool. You can optionally dust the top of your sweet beet cake with powdered sugar before serving.

Sweet courgette cake

Ingredients:
- Courgettes 300 g
- flour 250 g
- Almond flour 100 g
- Eggs 3
- Corn seed oil 200 ml
- Sugar 250 g
- Sweet baking powder 1 sachet
- Vanilla bean

Wash the courgettes, trim the ends, and shred them using a big hole grater before making the sweet zucchini cake. After beating the entire eggs and sugar together until frothy, stir in the 00 flour, almond or hazelnut flour, vanilla bean seeds, and well-sifted yeast. Incorporate the seed oil and thoroughly mix before adding the grated courgettes.

After thoroughly mixing, transfer the batter into a cake pan measuring 24 by 26 cm, covering it with parchment paper if desired. Test the cooked courgette cake with a toothpick after baking it for around 60 minutes at 180°C. After the first 40 minutes of cooking, if the surface gets too black, cover it with aluminum foil. Before transferring the zucchini cake, allow it to cool. Garnish it with powdered sugar!

Apple pie

Ingredients:
- Apples (700 g clean) 930 g
- Sugar 200 g
- flour 250 g
- Butter 100 g

- Whole milk (at room temperature) 150 g
- Eggs (at room temperature) 2
- Lemons 1
- Baking powder for sweets 16 g
- Cinnamon powder ½ tsp
- Salt up to a pinch

TO SPRAY

- Icing sugar to taste

First, melt the butter in a saucepan and set it aside to create the apple pie. Grate the zest of the lemon and squeeze the juice to yield around 30 g. Set aside the zest and juice. After the apples are peeled and the core removed, split them into four pieces and then cut each section into slices. To keep the apples from going black, put them in a basin and pour the lemon juice over them. Next, mix the baking powder and the 00 flour by sieving them together.

Next, transfer half of the sugar dose and the eggs into a large bowl. While using the electric whisk, begin whisking and gradually add the sugar. Add a little amount of salt as soon as the mixture begins to lighten, and beat the mixture until a frothy dough forms. Add the melted butter that has been brought back to room temperature at this point. Add the grated lemon zest and ground cinnamon for flavor. Subsequently, keep whisking while gradually adding the sifted flour and baking powder. Reduce the electric whisks' speed and pour the room-temperature milk flush after the powders are fully combined. The dough is ready when the milk is fully integrated; cease whipping. Pour the apples into the dough after draining them in a sieve to get rid of the lemon juice. To thoroughly combine them, gently stir from bottom to top. Pour the mixture into a cake tin with a 22-cm diameter after greasing and dusting it with sugar. When the cake is ready to be baked, bake it for around 55 minutes at 180 ° in a static oven that has been warmed.

Once cooked, remove from the oven and allow to cool. After dusting the cake with icing sugar, proceed to serve it.

Paradise cake

Ingredients:
- Light butter 170 g
- Icing sugar 170 g
- Sugar 40 g
- Salt up to 2,5 g
- Potato starch 70 g
- Sweet baking powder 3 g
- flour 100 g
- Vanilla bean
- Yolks 80 g
- Whole eggs 100 g
- ½ lemon zest
- Orange peel ½

TO SPREAD THE CAKE
- Icing sugar to taste

In a bowl, first sift together the starch, flour, and yeast. Grate half of the orange and lemon zest, add the pulp from half of the vanilla bean, and chunk up the butter in a different bowl. Begin by combining the icing sugar with the vanilla-flavored butter using an electric whisk. Add the 80 g of yolks (about four medium egg yolks) once the mixture has taken on a soft, airy consistency. Next, add the salt and keep whisking the mixture with the electric whisk until a creamy consistency is achieved.

Set aside. Pour the two whole eggs and the granulated sugar into a different bowl. Beat everything together with an electric whisk. Once the egg and sugar mixture is foamy, mix it with the bowl containing the yolks, butter, and sugar in turns.

Next, carefully stir in sugar and a small amount of the egg mixture. Next, include a portion of the powders and mix further. Once more, work with the liquid portion, and then, after you're done, use the powders. Take a 24 cm diameter mold, dust and butter it, then fill it with the paradise cake batter. Until the surface is uniform, level it with. For 45 to 50 minutes, bake the paradise cake in a static oven that has been prepared to 170 degrees. If the cake starts to color too much after 30 minutes, cover it with aluminum foil and keep cooking. When it's done (always test with a toothpick), remove from the oven and let cool for about 20 minutes before inverting onto a platter. After carefully removing the mold, give it about an hour to cool completely. After it cools, dust the surface with icing sugar until it forms a uniform layer. The cake is prepared!

Yogurt soft cake

Ingredients:
- Low-fat yogurt 320 g
- Eggs (about 4) 220 g
- Room temperature butter 150 g
- Sugar 200 g
- flour 250 g

- Corn starch (cornstarch) 80 g
- Untreated lemon zest 1
- Salt up to a pinch
- Baking powder (1 sachet) 16 g

Slice the butter into cubes and allow it to soften before making the yogurt cake. After that, add it to the sugar in the bowl of a planetary mixer and blend for at least ten minutes. After the mixture becomes creamy, add the eggs one at a time, letting each one fully integrate before adding the next. After you've mixed in all of the eggs, add the yogurt and a little amount of salt while continuing to whisk. Using a spatula, lightly mix the dough after grating in the zest of one lemon. Mix the flour, yeast, and cornstarch in a bowl, then gradually add the mixture to the dough by sieving it. Use a spatula to mix the mixture thoroughly and gently, turning it from bottom to top so as not to break it apart.

Pour the mixture into a cake tin that has been greased and floured, then use a spatula to level the top. Bake for approximately 50 minutes at 175 ° in a static preheated oven (cook at 155 ° for 40 minutes if using a fan oven). Always use a toothpick to check if the cake is baked correctly. After the cake is done, take it out of the oven, let it cool, then take it out of the form and let it cool fully. Your light cake is now prepared for consumption!

CHAPTER 7

RECIPES FOR SNACK

Tongues of cat

Ingredients:
- Soft butter, ointment 50 g
- Icing sugar 60 g
- Egg whites 50 g
- Flour 0 50 g

Transfer the soft butter into a bowl in order to prepare the cat's tongues. Utilizing a spatula, add the icing sugar and stir. Actually, there won't be a need to mount this bulk. Add the egg whites and stir until the mixture is creamy again. Once more, mix after adding the flour until a soft mass forms. Spoon the dough into a sac-à-poche using a smooth nozzle measuring 10 mm. Cut around 15 sticks, each measuring about 10 cm in length, using a dripping pan fitted with parchment paper. Bake for roughly 8 minutes at 190° in a convection oven that has been preheated. The cat's tongues will be prepared at this point. Take them out of the oven, and if you would rather shape them differently than normal while they are still hot, move them to a rolling pin and allow to cool. In this manner, a wave-like shape will result. Otherwise, simply allow them to cool in the pan to get a straight form. Transfer to a serving plate and serve, or use to create a dessert that lets your creativity run wild.

Cookies with two ingredients

Ingredients:
- Ripe bananas (approx. 2) 300 g
- Cereal muesli 100 g
- Dark chocolate chips (optional) to taste

The two-ingredient biscuits are made by first adding the cereal muesli to a bowl, then peeling, slicing, and removing the filaments from the bananas. Place the bananas in a potato masher, then pour the pureed bananas into the bowl containing the cereal muesli. After giving the mixture a quick stir, feel free to include the chocolate droplets. Next, take a dripping pan, cover it with parchment paper, and distribute tiny piles of dough with a spoon. Be careful to compact the biscuits firmly and space them apart to prevent sticking during cooking. Stir again with the spoon to disperse the drops equally. The biscuits will be firmer and retain their shape if you let them rest in the freezer for ten minutes. After that, bake them for fifteen minutes at 180 ° in a preheated static oven (or for roughly ten minutes in a convection oven at 160 °). When cooked, remove the biscuits from the oven and cool them on a wire rack by carefully removing them from the pan with a spatula. Your biscuits with just two ingredients are prepared for consumption!

Cookies with chocolate chips

Ingredients:

- Chocolate drops 100 g
- flour 500 g
- Eggs (medium) 2
- Brown sugar 200 g
- Vanilla bean 1
- Baking soda 3 g
- Salt up to a pinch
- Butter (softened) 180 g

Waffle

Ingredients:

- flour 280 g
- Butter 220 g
- Medium eggs, at room temperature 6
- Baking powder for cakes 2 g
- Sugar 180 g
- Vanilla bean 1
- Salt up to 1 tsp

TO SEAL

- Fresh fruit to taste
- Maple syrup to taste
- Icing sugar to taste

Melt the butter in a pan and set aside to cool before making the waffles. While waiting, crack the room-temperature eggs into a basin and whisk them softly. Add the sugar and stir one more. Pour the flour and yeast straight into the bowl, then stir in the salt. Eliminate any lumps from the mixture by thoroughly mixing in the granules.

After it has cooled, carefully incorporate the melted butter into the bowl by adding small amounts at a time. Now cut open the vanilla pod and use a knife to scrape out the seeds. Add the seeds to the mixture and stir again until a thick, uniform consistency forms. The dough should rest in the refrigerator for an hour after being covered with plastic wrap in the bowl. Allow the dough to come back to room temperature after the rest period. In the interim, preheat the waffle iron. Once the plate is heated, apply a thin layer of melted butter on it and use a ladle to fill the honeycomb-shaped mold all the way to the top. Shut off the plate and cook for approximately 7 to 8 minutes (check the doneness after 2.3 minutes). Once the waffles have turned a gorgeous golden hue, carefully remove them from the pan and place them on a dish by opening the lid.

Garnish the waffles with icing sugar, fresh fruit, and maple syrup, as per your preference.

Praline almonds

Ingredients:
- Almonds 150 g
- Sugar 120 g
- Water 35 g

Prepare a dripping pan by lining it with parchment paper before beginning to make the praline almonds. Now grab a pan and fill it with room-temperature water, sugar, and almonds. After turning on the medium-low heat, begin mixing. The water and sugar mixture will be extremely liquid at first, but as it begins to boil, it will eventually crystallize and surround the almonds with a patina. Now turn down the heat a little bit and keep stirring until the sugar begins to caramelize. After the almonds have browned, spread them out on a baking dish covered with parchment paper. As the almonds cool, break them apart with your hands to keep them from sticking together. You may now savor your praline almonds!

Candied ginger

Ingredients:
- Water to taste
- Fresh ginger to clean 450 g

FOR SECOND COOKING
- Boiled ginger 160 g
- Sugar 160 g

- Water 100 g
- Salt up to 1 tsp

TO SEAL
- Sugar to taste

After peeling, chop the ginger into tiny, two-centimeter pieces. Put the ginger in a pan, cover it fully with water, and boil it for about half an hour. After the ginger has boiled, strain it, put it in a saucepan, and then add the salt, sugar, and 100 grams of water. Cook, stirring, over medium heat for 20 minutes. Once the cooking time is up, remove the heat source and allow the mixture to cool. Place parchment paper on a baking sheet and dust the surface with sugar. Pour the cooled ginger, divide the pieces, and then top with additional sugar. To improve the sugar's adhesion, gather the ginger in foil. After allowing it to cool, store the candied ginger in a jar and eat it as a snack.

Apple chips

Ingredients:
- Red Apples 500 g
- Sugar 150 g
- Water 200 g
- Lemon juice 1

Melt the sugar and water in a saucepan over low heat to begin creating the syrup. After transferring the syrup to a baking dish and allowing it to cool, squeeze a lemon and stir its juice into the syrup. This will stop the apples from turning black when they are sliced. After washing, cut out the cores, and thinly slice the apples (you may help yourself with a mandolin) until they are just a few millimeters thick. Once the syrup is ready, dip the apple slices into it. After draining, transfer them to pans lined with parchment paper. Dry them in an 80 degree fan oven for at least 5 or 6 hours, rotating them halfway through with a small knife. It's likely that the apple chips will remain soft to the touch even after baking for five or six hours, but don't worry this is only the result of the heat. They will become crunchy and ready to munch as soon as they cool!

Spelled crackers

Ingredients:
- Spelled flour 250 g
- Dry white wine 80 g
- Extra virgin olive oil 50 g
- Cold butter butter 25 g
- Thyme 3 sprigs
- Salt up to 6 g

TO BRUSH AND CONDITION
- Water to taste
- Coarse salt (optional) 8 g
- Poppy seeds 5 g
- Sunflower seeds 5 g
- Flax seeds 5 g

In order to make the spelled crackers, first place the spelled flour in a big basin, then add the fresh thyme and fine salt and stir thoroughly. Working with your hands, incorporate the butter into the flour mixture, followed by the white wine and olive oil. Once the dough is compact, place it on a surface that has been lightly floured and use a rolling pin to spread it out until you have a sheet that is roughly 28 by 24 cm and has a thickness of approximately 4-5 mm. Using a fork, prick the dough and divide it into squares that are around 4 cm square on each side.

Now, combine the flax, sunflower, poppy, and flaxseeds in a small bowl along with the coarse salt.

Gently press with your hands to ensure that the coarse salt and seed mixture sticks to the surface once you have sprinkled it on. After transferring the dough pieces to a parchment paper-lined dripping pan, lightly mist them with water. Bake on the middle shelf of a static oven that has been warmed to 170° for about 25 minutes. After cooking, allow them to cool before serving the spelled crackers as a midday snack!

Pasta balls with honey

Ingredients:
FOR THE MIXTURE
- 250 g of 00 flour
- 4 g of baking powder
- 2 medium eggs
- 20 g of granulated sugar
- 30 g of melted butter
- Zest of half a lemon
- The zest of half an orange
- A pinch of salt

TO DECORATE
- 150 g of honey
- 2 tablespoons of granulated sugar
- colored sprinkles

Start by sifting the flour and yeast to prepare the dough for making the pasta balls in the oven. After adding the other ingredients, stir until a thick, uniform mixture is formed. Now, divide the dough into five to six sections, and use each portion to form a thin cylinder that is about one to two centimeters in diameter. Slice the cylinders into pieces that are approximately 1 centimeter thick, then put them on a sizable pan with parchment paper that is slightly ajar on top. Give them 20 minutes to rest in the fridge. Bake the pasta for 10 to 11 minutes at 180 degrees in a preheated oven, or until it turns golden.

Meanwhile, bring the honey and sugar to a simmer in a saucepan. Pour the cooked pasta balls and candied fruit into the saucepan once the sugar has melted fully. Mix thoroughly until all of the honey and other ingredients are incorporated into the biscuits. Transfer to a serving platter and allow to cool. They're prepared to be eaten now!

Biscuits with almonds

Ingredients:

- 2 eggs
- 170 g of granulated sugar
- 280 g of 00 flour
- ½ teaspoon of baking soda
- 40 g of soft butter
- 70 g of shelled and unpeeled almonds
- 1 tbsp honey
- 1 yolk to brush

To prepare the biscuits, begin by combining the two whole eggs with granulated sugar in a boule and using an electric mixer for a limited period of time. To get a grainy dough, add the flour and baking soda and stir. Incorporate the honey, butter, and whole almonds. Create a dough by kneading the material.

Split the dough in half and form a loaf with each half using your lightly floured hands. Place both of them on a parchment paper-lined baking sheet, then brush each with egg yolk. Bake for 20 minutes at 190° in a preheated oven.

Take them out, give them a few minutes to rest, and then cut each strand into diagonal slices that are approximately a centimeter thick to create biscuits. Bake the biscuits at 200° for a further 5 minutes to brown them. When they are cool enough to handle, take them out of the oven and serve.

CHAPTER 8

DRINKS&SHAKES

Golden milk

Ingredients:
- Water 130 g
- Turmeric powder 40 g
- Black pepper 1 pinch

FOR A GOLDEN MILK CUP
- Vegetable milk (almond or soy) 150 g
- honey 1 tbsp

Turmeric paste is the first ingredient you must make in order to make golden milk. Add a little pinch of pepper to a pot filled with water, then bring to a boil. Add the turmeric powder and switch off the heat as soon as the water boils. Mix until a thick, granular paste forms. Lastly, move the paste made from turmeric into a jar so you can preserve it there. Proceed to the next step:

making your golden milk. Heat the vegetable milk in a pot until it boils, then pour it into a jar, add a teaspoon of turmeric paste, sweeten with honey, and screw on the lid. All set for your milk with gold hues!

Banana milkshake

Ingredients:
- Bananas 300 g
- Ice 60 g
- Cinnamon sticks 2 g
- Whole milk 150 g

We begin by chopping the bananas into chunks and adding them to the mixer to make the banana smoothie. Incorporate the cinnamon, a moderate amount of ice cubes, and room temperature milk. Run the mixer until a creamy, thick mixture comes out. After that, pour it into the cups and garnish with a few cinnamon sticks. It's time for the milkshake.

Yogurt smoothie

Ingredients:
- Yogurt 250 g
- Lime juice (about 1) 13 g
- Pulp melon 420
- Pulp peaches 350

It will take around three peaches to wash, peel, and remove the core. Next, chop the peaches into coarse bits and set them aside. The melon is now ready to be cut into pieces. Cut it in half, take out the seeds, and peel it. Squeeze the lime after cutting it in half. Gather the extracted juice in a glass and set it away. Now place the melon in a blender. After adding the yogurt and lime juice, shut off the blender and turn it on. Blend the mixture until it becomes creamy. It's time for your yogurt smoothie!

Almond milk

Ingredients:
- Peeled almonds 200 g
- Water 1 l
- Acacia honey 85 g

Almonds should be soaked for at least an hour in a dish filled with 500 g of water before making almond milk. After an hour, add the remaining 500 g of water and honey to a mixer along with the almonds and water. Mix all ingredients together until a smooth cream is achieved, then pour the mixture through a fine-mesh strainer and store in the refrigerator, wrapped with plastic wrap, for at least one hour. You can serve your almond milk at room temperature or cold.

Homemade tropical fruit juice

Ingredients:

- 450 g of pineapple
- 250g mango
- 2 oranges
- 1 grapefruit
- 1.2 liters of water
- 100g of sugar

Peel the mango and cut it into cubes first. Cut the pineapple in half, then in four halves after removing the ends. Make the cubes pineapple-shaped and remove the hard center section. Next, squeeze the juice from the grapefruit and orange. After that, add the fruit cubes and citrus juice to the saucepan with the water and sugar, and cook for fifteen minutes. After using a hand blender for 15 minutes to purée the ingredients, place them in glass jars that have been sterilized. Once the jars are closed, place them in the refrigerator to allow them to chill. They're now prepared for tasting!

Non-alcoholic melon cocktail

Ingredients:

- 1 untreated lemon
- 20 grams of sugar
- 2 slices of melon
- 2 slices of white melon
- 400 milliliters of carbonated mineral water

Peel and rinse the lemon, being careful not to discard the zest. Cut the lemon in halves, squeeze off the juice, and strain the liquid through a sieve.

Place the lemon zest and the strained juice in a saucepan with 20 grams of sugar. Stirring constantly, cook everything on low heat for 2 minutes. After filtering, allow the resulting syrup to cool. Remove the seeds and white filaments from both the melon and the white melon after peeling them. Cut the melons' pulp into tiny pieces. Blend the melon chunks in the blender until a homogenous mixture is achieved. To the melon smoothie, add the syrup that was previously made. Gradually blend in the carbonated mineral water with your non-alcoholic drink. Blend once more, then transfer to a container or cocktail glasses and store in the fridge. Allow them to cool for thirty minutes. When you're done, add straws and melon slices to the glasses as you choose. While still extremely fresh, serve the non-alcoholic melon drink.

Smoothie cheesecake

Ingredients:
- Lean cottage cheese 250 g
- Fresh liquid cream 250 g
- Icing sugar 30 g
- Strawberries 280 g
- Yellow peaches 380 g

In order to prepare the cheesecake smoothie, wash the strawberries and peach first. Then, cut the peach into pieces and peel it. Put the pieces in the glass mixer and blend until a puree is achieved. Apply the same procedure to the strawberries: take off the green stems, chop them into small pieces, and put them in the glass mixer to blend until a puree is achieved. To create a homogenous cream, transfer the ricotta into a bowl, then mix in ¾ of the new liquid cream and the icing sugar. Use an immersion mixer to integrate everything together. Finally, pour in the remaining fresh liquid cream and stir. Create a cheesecake smoothie now. Use glasses that hold roughly 70 cl. The smoothie consists of layers of fruit puree and ricotta cream alternately. Pour the first layer of cream, then use your hands to slightly stir the glass to spread the cream evenly across the bottom. Next, pour a layer of ricotta cream, and finally top with the puree of strawberries or peaches.

Present your delicious cheesecake smoothie!

Apple cider

Ingredients:
- 700 grams of apples
- 50 grams of sugar
- 100 ml of water
- 1 orange
- 1 lemon
- 2 cloves
- 1 cinnamon stick
- 1 fresh ginger

Cut the orange into pieces, squeeze off the juice, and set aside to start making the apple cider. Proceed similarly with the lemon. Now wash the apples, peel them, and cut out the core. Now chop the apples into cubes and process them in a blender to extract the juice. Strain the mixture through a sieve. To combine all the tastes, add the sugar now, along with the juices of the orange and lemon. Add the cinnamon, cloves, and fresh ginger now, and simmer for ten minutes. Your apple cider is ready once the ten minutes have passed and everything has been filtered.

Chai latte

Ingredients:
- 200 ml milk
- 200 ml water
- 2 black tea bags
- 1 pinch of cinnamon
- 1 pinch of cardamom
- 2 ginger sticks
- 1 teaspoon maple syrup

First, fill a saucepan with water and bring it to a boil. After the water reaches a boiling point, switch off the burner and add the spices and tea bags. Take out the tea bags after a few minutes and let them steep for an additional four. Meanwhile, add milk and a teaspoon of maple syrup to another saucepan. Mix thoroughly with a wooden spoon until all of the syrup has been drained. Now that the infusion has been added, thoroughly stir the milk to combine the flavors. All set!

Fruit and yogurt cocktails

Ingredients:
- 25 gr of strawberries
- 25 gr of raspberries
- 125 ml of cold milk
- 125 ml of Cold Natural Yogurt
- 1 Teaspoon Rose Water
- 1/2 teaspoon of light honey

To prepare, place the milk, yogurt, raspberries, strawberries, and rose water in a blender. Blend for approximately 30 seconds, making sure all of the ingredients are properly combined.

Transfer into a tall glass, stir, and then stir in the honey. Serve right away after decorating with strawberry slices or a mint sprig.

CONCLUSION

An inflammatory condition affecting the stomach and digestive tract is called GERD. The primary causes of this issue include inadequate diet, impaired digestion, insufficient sleep, and an unhealthy way of living. Acid reflux can be brought on by weight gain and other medical issues. Heartburn and the sensation that food is returning from the stomach are symptoms of GERD. The first line of treatment for GERD is eating the right foods, exercising, and trying to lose weight while adhering to a balanced diet. If left untreated, it might lead to more severe health issues like cancer or ulcers. You must make certain lifestyle adjustments, such as eating smaller meals rather than larger ones, exercising regularly, cutting back on the amount of spicy and fried foods you eat, and so on, in order to get rapid GERD relief. Eating a healthy, organic diet can help prevent and treat

GERD during its early stages. Additionally, have a sufficient medical examination; this will enable you to determine the severity of the issue. Speak with your family physician and pay attention to the precautions and treatment suggestions that they have made. The first thing you should do to treat GERD is this. This book has a number of organic and healthful recipes that will enable you to finally enjoy delicious meals and relief from acid reflux symptoms.